HOME WORK OUT FOR OLDER WOMEN

The Senior Strength Training Guide to Help Improve Flexibility Mobility Energy and Balance

Emily Richard

Copyright ©2024 Emily Richard

All Rights Reserved

TABLE OF CONTENT

HOME WORKOUTS NUMEROUS BENEFITS AND SIGNIFICANT IMPORTANCE FOR OLDER WOMEN:

1. Convenience:

Home workouts allow older women to exercise at their own convenience, eliminating the need to travel to a gym or fitness class. This flexibility makes it easier to incorporate regular exercise into their daily routine.

2. Comfort and Privacy:

Exercising at home provides a comfortable and private environment where older women can feel at ease, especially if they're self-conscious about working out in public settings.

This privacy can enhance motivation and confidence.

3. Safety:

Home workouts reduce the risk of accidents and injuries associated with navigating unfamiliar gym equipment or participating in crowded fitness classes.

Older women can exercise in a familiar and controlled environment, minimizing the chance of falls or strain.

4. Tailored Workouts:

Home workouts allow older women to customize their exercise routine to suit their individual needs, preferences, and fitness level. They can choose exercises that target specific areas of concern or accommodate any physical limitations they may have.

5. Cost-Effectiveness:

Avoiding gym memberships or class fees can save older women money in the long run.

Home workouts can be done with minimal or no equipment, utilizing bodyweight exercises or affordable fitness tools like resistance bands or yoga mats.

6. Flexibility:

Older women can adapt their home workouts to fit their schedule, whether they prefer to exercise in the morning, afternoon, or evening.

They can also modify the duration and intensity of their workouts based on their energy levels and other commitments.

7. Improved Health:

Regular home workouts contribute to improved overall health and well-being for older women.

Physical activity helps maintain muscle strength, flexibility, and bone density, reducing the risk of age-related conditions such as osteoporosis and sarcopenia.

8. Mental Health Benefits:

Exercise has been shown to have positive effects on mental health by reducing stress, anxiety, and symptoms of depression.

Home workouts provide older women with a convenient way to relieve tension and improve mood without leaving the comfort of their home.

9. Social Connection:

Home workouts can be a shared activity for older women and their partners, friends, or family members, promoting social interaction and bonding. Exercising together can enhance motivation and accountability while fostering a sense of community.

10. Long-Term Independence:

By maintaining an active lifestyle through home workouts, older women can improve their mobility, balance, and functional ability, ultimately supporting long-term independence and quality of life as they age.

In summary, home workouts offer older women a convenient, safe, and customizable way to stay active, improve health, and enhance overall well-being.

Regular exercise at home can contribute to a happier, healthier, and more fulfilling life in the golden years.

EXERCISE SAFETY TIPS:

1. Contact with a Healthcare Professional: Before beginning any new workout routine, particularly if you have pre-existing health issues or medical conditions, contact with your healthcare practitioner to verify that the activities you choose are safe and appropriate for you.

2. Start slowly and Gradually: Begin with workouts that are appropriate for your present fitness level, gradually increasing intensity or time as you gain comfort and confidence. Avoid pushing yourself too hard, especially when beginning out.

3. Warm-Up and Cool Down: Always start your workout with a mild warm-up to prepare your muscles and joints for action, and finish with a cool-down to help your body recuperate. This may involve gentle stretching and deep breathing exercises.

4. Listen to Your Body: Pay attention to how you feel when exercising. If you develop discomfort, dizziness, shortness of breath, or any other strange symptoms, stop right away and get medical attention if necessary. It's critical to discern between discomfort from exercise and pain from an injury.

5. Maintain Good Form and technique throughout workouts to reduce the chance of injury and enhance efficacy. If you're unclear how to do a specific exercise correctly, see a skilled fitness professional.

6. Stay Hydrated: Drink water before, during, and after your workout to stay hydrated, especially if you sweat a lot. Dehydration can impair performance and increase the likelihood of injury.

7. Adapt workouts as Needed: Don't be afraid to adapt workouts to meet your specific requirements and talents. This might include employing props or equipment for support, changing range of motion, or selecting more appropriate workouts for your body.

8. Create a Safe Exercise Environment: Make sure your workout area is clear of risks and impediments that might cause trips or falls. Use sturdy furniture or equipment for support, and consider adding non-slip mats or carpets to prevent falls.

9. Dress appropriately: Wear comfortable, breathable clothing and supportive footwear according to the sort of exercise you're doing. Avoid wearing loose or tight apparel that might limit movement or cause harm.

10. Listen to Your Body: Remember that rest is an important part of any fitness plan. Allow your body enough time to recuperate between exercises, and don't be afraid to take pauses or change the intensity as needed. To maintain a long-term fitness habit, prioritize self-care and pay attention to your body's cues.

15 MOBILITY AND WARM-UP EXERCISES.

1. Neck Rolls:

Stand or sit tall, keeping your shoulders relaxed.

Slowly lower your chin to your chest and turn your head in a circular motion, bringing your ear to your shoulder before moving to the opposite side.

Repeat both directions.

2. Shoulder Rolls:

Stand tall, arms at your sides.

Roll your shoulders forward in a circular motion, elevating them to your ears, then back down.

Reverse the action by rolling your shoulders backward.

3. Arm Circles:

Extend your arms out to the sides, shoulder height.

Make tiny circles with your arms, gradually increasing the size of each circle.

After a few repetitions, flip orientations and draw circles in the opposite way.

4. Wrist Circles:

Extend your arms in front of you to shoulder height, palms facing down.

Create circles with your wrists, spinning clockwise and then counterclockwise.

5. Ankle Circles:

Sit on the edge of a chair, feet flat on the floor.

Lift one foot off the ground and spin your ankle in a circular manner, first clockwise, then anticlockwise.

Repeat with the other foot.

6. Hip Circles:

Stand with your feet hip-width apart, hands on your hips.

Circle your hips clockwise, then counterclockwise.

7. Knee Hugs:

Stand tall and bring one knee to your chest, clasping your hands around it.

Hold the posture for a few seconds before lowering your foot back down.

Repeat on the opposite knee.

8. Leg Swings (Front to Back):

Stand next to a wall or a solid surface for balance support.

Swing one leg forth and backward in a controlled manner while maintaining it straight.

Repeat with the opposite leg.

9. Leg Swings (Side to Side):

Stand next to a wall or a solid surface for balance support.

Swing one leg from side to side in a controlled manner while maintaining it straight.

Repeat with the opposite leg.

10. Knee Circles:

Stand with feet hip-width apart and hands on hips.

Bend one knee and draw circles by rotating it clockwise and then counterclockwise.

Repeat on the opposite knee.

11. Cat-Cow Stretch:

Begin on your hands and knees, placing your wrists precisely under your shoulders and your knees beneath your hips.

Inhale and arch your back, lowering your belly to the ground and rising your head and tailbone to the ceiling (Cow Pose).

Exhale while rounding your back, tucking your chin into your chest and bringing your belly button toward your spine (Cat Pose).

Repeat the sequence many times.

12. Standing Forward Fold:

Place your feet hip-width apart and tilt forward at the hips, reaching for the ground with your hands.

Bend your knees slightly if necessary, and allow your head and neck rest.

Hold the stretch for a few breaths before slowly rolling back to a standing position.

13. Side Stretch:

Stand with your feet hip width apart and your arms stretched overhead.

Grab your left wrist with your right hand and bend slightly to the right to stretch the left side of your body.

Hold the stretch for a few breaths before switching sides.

14. Torso Twist:

Stand with your feet hip-width apart and arms outstretched to the sides.

Twist your torso to the right, bringing your left hand across your body and touching your right hand.

Hold the stretch for a few breaths before twisting to the left and repeat.

15. March in Place:

Stand tall, feet hip-width apart.

Lift your knees to your chest one at a time, as if you were marching in place.

Pump your arms in sync with your legs to boost the intensity of the workout.

These mobility and warm-up exercises can help your body get ready for physical activity by boosting blood flow, improving flexibility, and lowering the chance of injury.

To improve your performance and enjoyment, incorporate them into your training program before moving on to more demanding activities.

15 STRENGTH TRAINING EXERCISES

Bodyweight Squats: Position your feet shoulder-width apart.

Bend your knees and push your hips back, just like you're sitting in a chair.

Maintain an upright posture with a straight back and chest.

Lower until your thighs are parallel to the ground, then push through your heels to go back to the starting position.

1. Wall Push-Ups:

Stand facing a wall, arms outstretched to shoulder height, palms flat against the wall.

Bend your elbows to lower yourself towards the wall while keeping your torso straight.

Straightening your arms will help you return to your starting posture.

2. Chair Squats:

Stand in front of a chair, feet hip-width apart. Lower your body by bending your knees and pulling your hips back, as if you were ready to sit in the chair.

Keep your chest high and your weight on your heels.

Touch the chair with your buttocks, then stand back up.

3. Chair Dips:

Sit on the edge of a strong chair, hands clutching the edge next to your hips.

Slide your buttocks off of the chair and move your feet forward. Bend your elbows to lower your body to the ground, then push back up to the starting position.

4. Bicep Curls:

Hold a dumbbell in each hand, stretch your arms down by your sides, palms facing forward.

Bend your elbows, keeping them close to your sides, and curl the weights towards your shoulders.

Slowly lower the weights back down with control.

5. Triceps kickbacks:

Hold a dumbbell in each hand and tilt forward at the hips while maintaining your back flat.

 Bend your elbows and bring the weights to your sides.

Stretch your arms straight back, squeezing your triceps at the top, then return to the beginning position.

6. Seated Leg Extensions:

Sit in a chair, feet flat on the floor, and a dumbbell on each thigh. Lift one leg straight ahead of you, squeezing your quadriceps at the top, then drop it back down.

 Repeat on the opposite side.

7. Seated Shoulder Press:

Sit on a chair with one dumbbell in each hand, palms facing forward and elbows bent at 90 degrees.

Press the weights above until your arms are completely extended, then drop them to shoulder height.

8. Standing Calf Raises:

Stand with your feet hip-width apart and your hands resting on a stable surface for balance if necessary.

As high as you can on the balls of your feet, then return to the ground.

9. Standing Hip Abductions:

Stand with your feet together, holding onto a solid surface for balance if necessary.

Lift one leg to the side while maintaining it straight, then drop it back down with control.

Repeat on the opposite side.

10. Deadlifts with Dumbbells:

Hold a dumbbell in each hand, arms outstretched in front of your thighs.

Keep your back straight and your knees slightly bent, then lean forward at the hips while lowering the weights to the ground.

Keep the weights close to your body and squeeze your glutes and hamstrings to return to the beginning position.

11. Bent over Rows:

Hold a dumbbell in each hand, palms facing you.

Bend your knees slightly and lean forward from the hips, maintaining your back flat.

Bend your elbows and pull the dumbbells up towards your ribcage before lowering them with control.

12. Reverse Lunges:

Stand with your feet together, holding a dumbbell at either side. Take a step back with one foot, dropping your back knee to the ground while keeping your front knee bent at a 90° angle.

Push through your front heel to return to the starting position, then repeat on the opposite side.

13. Plank:

Begin in a push-up posture, with your hands precisely under your shoulders and your body in a straight line from head to heels.

Engage your core muscles and keep this position as long as possible while inhaling deeply.

14. Russian Twists:

Sit on the floor with your knees bent and your feet flat.

Lean back slightly and slowly then raise your feet off the ground.

Hold a dumbbell in both hands and rotate your body to the right, then left, maintaining your core engaged and your back straight.

These workouts target different muscle groups and may be modified in terms of weight and intensity to meet your fitness level.

Always warm up before beginning your workout and cool down afterwards to avoid injury and enhance healing.

If you're new to strength training, see a fitness professional to guarantee appropriate form and technique.

15 FLEXIBILITY EXERCISES:

1. Sit on the floor, one leg straight in front of you and the other bent. Reach for your toes on the outstretched leg while maintaining your back straight.

 Hold the stretch for 15-30 seconds and then swap legs.

2. Quadriceps Stretch:

 Stand tall and elevate one foot towards your buttocks, holding your ankle with your hand.

Keep your knees together and your thighs aligned.

Hold the stretch for just 15-30 seconds and then swap legs.

3. Calf Stretch:

Stand facing a wall, hands against it at shoulder height.

Step one foot back and drive the heel into the ground, keeping the rear leg straight.

Lean slightly forward until you feel a stretch in the calf of your rear leg.

Hold for just 15-30 seconds and then swap legs.

4. Butterfly Stretch:

Sit on the floor, soles of your feet together, knees bent out to the sides.

 Hold on to your feet and softly press your knees into the ground with your elbows.

Hold the stretch for about 15 to 30 seconds.

5. Seated Forward Bend:

Sit on the floor, legs straight in front of you, feet flexed.

Reach towards your toes while maintaining your back straight.

Hold the stretch for 15-30 seconds, concentrating on extending the spine.

6. Trunk Rotation Stretch:

Sit on the floor with your legs straight ahead of you.

Bend one knee and cross it over the opposing leg, with the foot flat on the floor.

Twist your body towards the bent knee, gently pressing your opposing elbow into the outside of the knee.

Hold for few seconds (15-30) seconds and then swap sides.

7. Shoulder Stretch:

Stand tall and extend one arm across your body, gently pressing the opposing hand on your chest.

Hold for 15-30 seconds and then swap arms.

8. Chest Opener Stretch:

Stand tall with your arms stretched behind you and clasped together. Lift your arms slightly and open your chest, pressing your shoulder blades together.

Hold for 15–30 seconds.

9. Neck Stretch:

Sit or stand tall, shoulders relaxed.

Tilt your head to one side and bring your ear near your shoulder.

Hold for just 15-30 seconds and then swap sides.

10. Wrist Flexor Stretch:

Extend one arm in front of you, palm facing down.

Using your opposite hand, gently push the fingers of the extended hand against your body until you feel a stretch in your wrist and forearm.

Hold for 15-30 seconds and then swap arms.

11. Wrist Extensor Stretch:

Extend one arm in front of you, palm up. Using your opposite hand, gently push the fingers of the extended hand to the floor until you feel a stretch in your wrist and forearm. Hold for 15-30 seconds and then swap arms.

12. Seated Spinal Twist:

Sit on the floor, legs straight in front of you.

Bend one knee and cross it over the opposing leg, with the foot flat on the floor.

Twist your torso towards the bent knee, using your opposing hand to support yourself.

Hold for just 15-30 seconds and then swap sides.

13. Ankle Circles:

Sit on the floor, legs straight in front of you.

Point your toes and draw circles with your ankles, first clockwise, then counterclockwise.

Repeat a few times and then swap feet.

14. Lateral Flexion Stretch:

Stand tall, feet hip-width apart, arms stretched overhead.

Reach one arm up and across to the other side, bending at the waist. Hold for just 15-30 seconds and then swap sides.

15. *Full Body Stretch:*

Stand tall, with your feet hip-width apart.

 Extend your arms above and reach for the ceiling, expanding your entire frame.

Hold for just 15-30 seconds and then release.

These flexibility exercises can help you improve your joint range of motion, relieve muscular tension, and increase general mobility.

Incorporate them into your daily routine to maintain and improve flexibility, promote good posture, and avoid injuries.

15. CARDIOVASCULAR EXERCISES

15 cardiovascular activities you may include in your fitness routine:

1. Walk briskly around your area or on a treadmill to increase your heart rate.

2. ***Jogging/Running:*** Exercise outside or on a treadmill to enhance cardiovascular fitness.

3. ***Cycling:*** Use a stationary bike or go outside to strengthen your lower body and increase cardiovascular endurance.

4. Perform jumping jacks to increase heart rate and stimulate the entire body.

5. ***High Knees:*** Increase heart rate and circulation by marching or jogging in place with raised knees.

6. ***Burpees:*** Squat, leap, and push-ups provide a full-body cardiovascular exercise.

7. **Jump Rope:** Exercises with a jump rope improve cardiovascular health and coordination.

8. ***Dancing:*** Dance to your favorite music in your living room to increase your heart rate and have fun.

9. ***Stair Climbing:*** Exercise your cardiovascular system by frequently ascending and descending steps, whether at home or on a machine.

10. ***Swim laps*** or do water aerobics to increase cardiovascular endurance and reduce joint impact.

11. ***Rowing***: A rowing machine simulates rowing a boat, providing a full-body cardiovascular exercise.

12. *Jump Squats:* Use an explosive jump at the top to enhance effort and raise heart rate.

13. *Kickboxing:* Improve cardiovascular fitness and learn self-defense methods by joining a training class or watching internet videos.

14. *Hiking:* Enjoy the outdoors and get a cardiovascular exercise on trails or in nature reserves.

15. *Circuit Training:* Combine cardiovascular workouts like jumping jacks, burpees, and mountain climbers in a fast sequence with minimum recovery.

Include these cardiovascular activities in your workout program to enhance heart health, boost endurance, and burn calories for general fitness and well-being.

Remember to begin gently, listen to your body, and keep hydrated during your workouts.

15 RELAXATION AND MIND-BODY PRACTICES.

15 relaxation and mind-body activities that can aid in relaxing, stress reduction, and general well-being:

1. Deep breathing

Exercises involve inhaling deeply through the nose, filling the lungs with air, and gently expelling through the mouth. Concentrate on your breathing to soothe your thoughts and relax your body.

2. Perform Progressive Muscle Relaxation (PMR)

By tensing and releasing each muscle group in your body, beginning with your toes and progressing to your head. This approach reduces bodily stress and promotes relaxation.

3. Guided Imagery:

Close your eyes and see yourself in a quiet setting, such a beach or forest. Visualize the sights, sounds, and sensations of this location to induce emotions of relaxation and calmness.

4. Body Scan Meditation:

Lie down in a comfortable posture and scan your body from head to toe. Bring awareness to each section and release any tension or discomfort you may feel.

5. Practice yoga positions

And stretches for relaxation, flexibility, and awareness. To build a sense of calm and present, try integrating your breath with movement.

6. Tai Chi:

Practice gentle, flowing motions to enhance balance, flexibility, and mental clarity. Tai Chi's meditation element helps to promote relaxation and stress reduction.

7. Qi Gong:

Use gentle movements, breath work, and visualization techniques to increase energy, reduce stress, and improve general well-being.

8. To practice mindfulness meditation, sit quietly and focus on the present now.

Observed your thoughts, feelings, and sensations without judgment.

Mindfulness meditation encourages relaxation and mental clarity.

9. Autogenic Training:

Use self-suggestion strategies to promote relaxation and well-being. Repeat words or affirmations about warmth, heaviness, and relaxation while concentrating on your breathing and physiological sensations.

10. Aromatherapy:

Use essential oils like lavender, chamomile, or bergamot to create a relaxing ambiance.

To achieve relaxing effects, diffuse the oils, add them to a bath, or use them physically.

11. Guided Meditation:

Use guided meditation recordings or apps to practice relaxation techniques, visualization, and mindfulness to reduce stress.

12. Journaling:

Record your thoughts, feelings, and experiences in a journal.

Journaling can help you process your feelings, develop insights, and reduce stress.

13. Nature Walks:

Enjoy leisurely walks in parks, forests, or gardens.

Connecting with nature helps soothe and center the mind and body.

14. Massage:

Get a professional massage or learn self-massage methods to relax muscles, relieve tension, and improve general well-being.

15. Relaxing Music:

Listen to calming music or nature sounds to encourage serenity and relaxation.

Pay attention to how the music makes you feel and allow yourself to relax.

Incorporate these relaxation and mind-body activities into your daily routine to relieve stress, promote relaxation, and improve your general well-being.

Experiment with several ways to see what works best for you, and remember to prioritize your own health and well-being.

15 DANCE WORKOUTS YOU WILL ENJOY:

1. Zumba:

Get a full-body exercise by dancing to lively Latin-inspired music in a class or through online videos.

2. Hip Hop Dance:

Practice rapid and dynamic dances to the rhythm of hip hop music.

3. Learn classic

Indian dance methods with a modern twist to immerse yourself in the bright world of Bollywood.

4. Take a Jazzercise class,

Which blends dancing, cardio, and strength training for an enjoyable and efficient exercise.

5. Learn seductive

And rhythmic salsa dancing routines to improve coordination and flexibility.

6. Ballet Fitness:

Use ballet-inspired moves and methods to enhance posture, strength, and flexibility.

7. African Dance:

Experience the vibrant cultural legacy of African dance via energetic motions and enticing rhythms that engage the entire body.

8. Learn belly dancing

To strengthen core muscles, enhance flexibility, and express oneself through dance.

9. Line Dancing:

Take a class or watch instructional videos to master coordinated dance sequences in lines or rows.

10. Flamenco Dance:

Master the complicated footwork, delicate arm motions, and dramatic expressions of this passionate and intense dance form.

11. Swing Dance:

Learn Lindy Hop, Charleston, and East Coast Swing for a dynamic dance experience inspired by the swing era of jazz music.

12. Samba Dance:

Learn the fast-paced footwork, hip motions, and addictive rhythms of this carnival-inspired dance.

13. Learn the rhythmic

And percussive moves of Irish step dancing, with sophisticated footwork and exciting music.

14. Ballroom Dancing:

Practice traditional ballroom dancing forms including foxtrot, waltz, tango, and cha-cha for a beautiful and graceful exercise.

15. Urban dance techniques

Like krumping, locking, popping, and breaking allow for artistic expression

While also providing cardio and strength workouts.

Choose one or more dance workouts that you enjoy and include them into your daily fitness program.

Dance is not only a terrific kind of exercise, but it's also a fun way to express yourself and interact with others.

15 CHAIR EXERCISES

1. Seated Marches:

Sit tall on the edge of a chair, feet level on the ground.

Lift one leg to your chest, then drop it, then repeat with the other knee.

Continue to alternate legs, as if you were marching in place.

2. Seated Leg Extensions:

Sit erect on a chair, feet flat on the floor.

Extend one leg straight in front of you and then drop it back down.

Repeat for the opposite leg.

Use ankle weights to enhance resistance.

3. Seated Toe Taps:

Sit on a chair with feet flat on the floor.

Lift your toes to the ceiling, then tap them back to the ground. Repeat a certain number of times.

4. Seated Knee Lifts:

Sit tall on the edge of a chair, feet flat on the floor.

 Lift one leg as high as possible toward your chest, then return it to the ground.

Repeat on the opposite knee.

5. Seated Heel Raises:

Sit erect on a chair, feet flat on the floor.

Lift your heels off the ground as high as possible, then drop them back down.

Repeat a certain number of times.

6. Side Leg Raises:

Sit on the edge of a chair, feet flat on the floor.

Lift one leg out to the side as far as you can, then drop it back down. Repeat for the opposite leg.

7. Seated Arm Circles:

 Sit erect on a chair, feet flat on the floor.

Extend your arms out to the sides, shoulder height.

Make tiny circles with your arms, gradually increasing the size of each circle.

8. Seated Shoulder Shrugs:

Sit tall on a chair, feet flat on the floor.

Lift your shoulders as far up towards your ears as you can, then bring them back down.

Repeat a certain number of times.

9. To do seated triceps dips,

Sit on the edge of a chair and grab the edge beside your hips.

Slide your buttocks off the chair, bend your elbows to drop your body to the ground, and then push yourself back up.

10. To perform a seated chest press,

Sit straight on a chair and hold a resistance band in each hand. Extend your arms straight in front of you, then press them together until your palms contact.

11. Seated Bicep Curls:

Sit tall on a chair with a resistance band beneath your feet and one in each hand.

Begin with your arms stretched down at your sides, then bend your elbows and curl the bands towards your shoulders.

12. Seated Leg Lifts:

Sit erect on a chair, feet flat on the floor.

Lift one leg straight in front of you and then drop it back down.

Repeat for the opposite leg.

13. Seated Crunches:

Sit on the edge of a chair, feet flat on the floor.

Place your hands behind your head, bend back slightly, and squeeze your chest toward your legs.

14. Seated Side Bends:

Sit tall in a chair and place your feet flat on the floor.

Place one hand behind your head and bend to the side, bringing your elbow to your hip.

Return to the starting position and repeat on the opposite side.

15. Seated Torso Twists:

Sit erect on a chair, feet flat on the floor.

Hold a lightweight item in both hands in front of you.

Twist your torso to one side, then back to the middle and twist the other way.

Repeat a certain number of times.

These chair exercises are ideal for people who have limited mobility or want to work out while sitting.

Incorporate them throughout your everyday regimen to increase your strength, flexibility, and general fitness.

www.ingramcontent.com/pod-product-compliance
Lightning Source LLC
Chambersburg PA
CBHW070756260726
48660CB00007B/3146